PAIN NO MORE

Menstrual cramps affect 90 percent of American women; it's estimated that, due to cramps, upwards of 140 million workhours are lost annually, as well as incalculable hours of quality of life. Now Dr. Susan Lark offers a self-help anti-cramp program that she has tested on hundreds of patients with permanently healthy results. This book helps women identify both their symptoms and their risk factors and shows them how to create an individualized program to alleviate those symptoms, including detailed information on diet, vitamins, minerals, herbs, stress reduction, breathing and physical exercises, yoga, acupressure and drug treatments.

ABOUT THE AUTHOR

Susan M. Lark, M.D. is one of the foremost authorities in the field of women's health care and preventive medicine. She has served on the clinical faculty of the Stanford University Medical School and has founded and directed many clinical programs in Northern California. In addition to maintaining a private practice, Dr. Lark has lectured throughout the United States and is the author of nine books on women's health issues.

Treating Menstrual Cramps Naturally

Effective natural solutions for discomforts most women face

Susan M. Lark, M.D.

Keats Publishing, Inc. New Canaan, Connecticut

Treating Menstrual Cramps Naturally is not intended as medical advice. Its intent is solely informational and educational. Please consult a health professional should the need for one be indicated.

TREATING MENSTRUAL CRAMPS NATURALLY

Copyright © 1996 by Susan M. Lark, M.D.

ISBN: 0-87983-712-8

Printed in the United States of America

Good Health Guides are published by
Keats Publishing, Inc.
27 Pine Street (Box 876)
New Canaan, Connecticut 06840-0876

Contents

INTRODUCTION

I have been a physician practicing women's health care and preventive medicine for almost two decades in the San Francisco area. I have worked with many thousands of women, combining traditional medical diagnostic and therapeutic techniques with a strong emphasis on the important role that self-care and a healthy lifestyle play in preventing disease and promoting wellness. I encourage my patients to be knowledgeable participants in their own healing process and health-care program, and I am continually impressed with how positively they respond to this approach.

I personally encountered the need for information during my teenage years and throughout my twenties when I suffered from severe menstrual cramps. I was anxious, irritable, bloated and obsessed by food cravings for many days of PMS prior to my period. Very little information was available on self-care treatments in the 1950s. I was instructed to take aspirin, a hot water bottle and go to bed until the cramps stopped. As a doctor-in-training I tried every medication possible — pain pills, muscle relaxants, antispasmodics—but nothing gave me anything but temporary relief.

Luckily, during my internship year, I spent time reading the latest medical research in my chosen specialty of obstetrics and gynecology. By chance I spotted an article on the successful treatment of breast lumps with vitamins. It was the first time I was exposed to the concept of nutrition as therapy, and it intrigued me that what I ate could affect my health. During the next few years I began to test a simple self-care program on myself. I made some dietary changes, cutting out sugar, fat, caffeine and junk foods, and I ate more whole grains, fresh vegetables and fruits. I started on a vitamin and mineral program based on the latest research in nutritional medicine, and I began to exercise regularly and practice stress management techniques.

I was amazed with the results. My symptoms began to diminish each month, and the quality of my life dramatically improved as my symptoms receded. After several years of self-care, my symptoms were entirely gone and have never come back. For the past 18 years my menstrual periods have been painless and symptom-free.

In the years since I put together my own treatment program, I have worked with many thousands of patients who have benefited from a self-care approach. I have spent years researching the use of diet, nutrition and many other lifestyle techniques that help prevent disease and benefit health. My goal has always been to give patients the information, education and resources they need to become healthier and maintain this state through healthy lifestyle practices. Most of my patients report that they feel much better within one or two menstrual cycles.

HOW TO USE THIS BOOK

I feel strongly that any woman interested in self-care should have access to the useful techniques I have developed over the years. I encourage each woman who reads this book to select from a wide variety of self-help treatment options. Included is information on diet, nutrition, vitamins, minerals and herbs, as well as programs on stress reduction, deep breathing, exercise, yoga and acupressure massage, all specifically designed to relieve symptoms of cramps and low back pain. I have found that results are much better with an individualized program; by overlapping treatments from various disciplines, most women find combinations that work best for them.

After seeing so many of my patients become healthier over time, I am a firm believer in the power of self-care. Read through the entire book first to familiarize yourself with the material. Making a monthly calendar (page 13) will help you evaluate your symptoms, and the treatment chart (page 20) will tell you which techniques to practice for your particular set of problems. These tools are quick and easy to use and will save you countless hours of experimentation on your own.

Try all the therapies listed under your particular symptoms, and you will find that some make you feel better than others. Establish a regimen that works for you and follow it every day. The feeling of wellness that can be yours with a self-help program will radiate out and enhance your whole life. Most of my patients tell me their lives have been positively transformed by following these beneficial self-help techniques.

WHAT ARE MENSTRUAL CRAMPS?

Menstrual cramps, or dysmenorrhea (medical term), are one of the most common health-care problems that women suffer during their reproductive years. It has been estimated that as many as 90 percent of women suffer from pain during their period, with the highest incidence in younger women in their teens to their thirties. At least 10 percent of younger women have symptoms so severe they are unable to function normally, forcing them to miss work and important social functions. These problems translate into billions of dollars of lost wages and job productivity, as well as a significant decrease in women's quality of life for several days each month. My gynecological textbook estimated that cramps cause the loss of 140 million work hours annually.

Despite this, cramps have traditionally been considered a "minor" ailment by the medical community. Doctors often treated women as though the problem were "all in their heads" or prescribed powerful painkilling drugs with significant side effects that did nothing to alleviate or prevent the problem. Luckily, the medical community's interest has increased over the past two decades, and researchers now understand more about what physiologically causes cramps. This had led to more effective drug treatments, as well as nutritional and lifestyle-related therapies.

THE NORMAL MENSTRUAL CYCLE

Each month the uterus prepares a thick, blood-rich cushion to nourish and house a fertilized egg. If pregnancy doesn't occur, the uterus cleanses itself, releasing the blood and tissue in the uterine lining (endometrium), so that a fresh buildup can occur the next month. The mechanism that regulates the buildup and shedding of the uterine lining is controlled by hormones—estrogen and progesterone, which are produced in the egg follicles in the ovaries. Estrogen output peaks during the first half of the cycle as the newly released egg is maturing. Progesterone output occurs after ovulation (release) of the mature egg has occurred during midcycle.

Estrogen and progesterone also stimulate the lining of the uterus. During the two weeks after menstruation, estrogen causes the uterine lining to triple in thickness by midcycle. Ovulation occurs, usually around day 14, and progesterone causes the lining to become more swollen. If the egg is fertilized, it may implant on the uterine wall, and progesterone continues to be secreted. If no fertilization occurs, progesterone levels decrease, and the uterine lining breaks down with menstruation.

TYPES AND CAUSES OF MENSTRUAL CRAMPS

There are two types of cramps: primary dysmenorrhea, in which pain is the main problem; and secondary dysmenorrhea, in which pain is a consequence of another health problem. Most women suffer from the first type, which is broken down into two subgroups: spasmodic and congestive.

Types of Cramps	Symptoms	Women Affected
Primary spasmodic dysmenorrhea	Severe viselike pain, backache, tightening & pain in inner thighs, nausea, vomiting, diarrhea, constipation, faintness, dizziness, fatigue, headaches	Teens Premenopausal wowen in their 40s and 50s
Primary congestive dysmenorrhea	Dull aching in low back & pelvis, bloating, weight gain, breast tenderness, headaches, irritability	Women in their 30s and 40s
Secondary dysmenorrhea	Pelvic & back pain, spotting, pain during or after sexual intercourse, fever, chills, puslike vaginal discharge, urinary frequency, bowel changes	Women in their 20s to 50s

Primary Spasmodic Dysmenorrhea (PSD)

PSD occurs when the uterine muscle and blood vessels that supply the uterus are tight and contracted. Blood circulation and oxygenation is diminished, metabolism of the uterus and pelvic muscles is decreased, and waste products of metabolism (carbon dioxide and lactic acid) build up, intensifying the pain and discomfort.

This type of cramping is linked to imbalances in the hormonal system. It may be the interplay between the two hormones that causes the tension and constriction; medical researchers don't know for sure. They do know that women who don't ovulate don't experience cramps, leading to the conclusion that progesterone must be present for cramping to occur.

Hormonelike chemicals called prostaglandins, derived from fatty acids in the diet, also affect muscle tension. There are many different types of prostaglandins. Series-two are linked to cramping, high blood pressure and irritable bowel syndrome and are found in animal fat — meat, dairy products and eggs. Series-one and series-three promote muscle relaxation and relieve cramps; they are found in vegetable and fish sources, including raw seeds (flax and pumpkin), nuts and certain fish (trout, mackerel and salmon). This is a good example of how food selection can affect the state of your health. Like progesterone, excessive prostaglandin production is linked to ovulation, increasing during the second half of the cycle and peaking with menstruation.

Primary Congestive Dysmenorrhea (PCD)

Symptoms of PCD are very different (see chart above). Excessive amounts of estrogen can worsen the symptoms, since estrogen increases fluid and salt retention in the body. Food allergies, especially to wheat and dairy products, and high-stress foods like alcohol, sugar and salt also contribute to congestive symptoms. When I put women on a salt-free, dairy-free, wheat-free diet, bloating decreases, as do abdominal discomfort and low back pain.

Other risk factors also contribute to both types of cramps:

Use of tampons	Childlessness (PSD)
Use of an IUD	Multiple pregnancies (PCD)
Bladder infections	Lack of exercise and poor posture
Vaginal yeast infections	Emotional stress

Secondary Dysmenorrhea

This type of uterine and low back pain is related to three underlying health problems: (1) fibroid tumors in the uterus, (2) pelvic inflammatory disease (PID) and (3) endometriosis.

Fibroid tumors, stimulated by estrogen, occur when the muscular tissue in the uterus grows excessively. They may expand with use of estrogen-dominated birth control pills, during pregnancy or in women who naturally secrete high levels of estrogen. If the tumors grow large enough to press on the bowel and bladder or outgrow their blood supply, they can worsen cramps, cause urinary frequency or bowel changes, excessive menstrual bleeding and pelvic discomfort to the point of necessitating a hysterectomy. In fact, fibroids account for many of the 750,000 hysterectomies performed yearly in the United States. Such tumors usually shrink after menopause when estrogen naturally decreases.

PID is an infection of the uterus, fallopian tubes or ovaries which must be treated immediately to prevent scarring and infertility. Symptoms include fever, chills, back pain, puslike vaginal discharge, pain during or after sexual intercourse and spotting. If untreated, this chronic pain can necessitate a hysterectomy.

Endometriosis occurs when pieces of the uterine lining (endometrium) grow in the pelvis outside the uterus. These tissues also respond to hormonal changes and bleed with the onset of menstruation, leading over time to scarring and inflammation of the pelvis. Pain is the most common symptom, which is heightened during menstruation and sexual intercourse.

Treatments for endometriosis vary depending on the woman's age, severity of symptoms and childbearing status. Supportive therapy includes antiprostaglandin medication, such as Motrin and Ponstel, and pregnancy is suggested, since it stops monthly menstruation (though women with endometriosis have higher levels of infertility because of structural damage). In some cases, physicians administer hormonal therapies, including birth control pills, that inhibit normal menstruation and growth of endometrial implants. In advanced cases, hysterectomy is advised.

EVALUATING YOUR SYMPTOMS

Begin by making a monthly calendar of your symptoms (photocopy the one below several times) and rate their severity, starting

Monthly Calendar of Menstrual Cramp Symptoms

Grade your symptoms as you experience them each month.
○ None ✓ Mild ◗ Moderate ● Severe

DAY OF CYCLE	1	2	3	4	5	6	7	8	9	10	11	12	13	14	15	16	17	18	19	20	21	22	23	24	25	26	27	28	29	30	31
Spasmodic Cramping																															
Viselike pelvic pain																															
Low back pain																															
Pain in inner thighs																															
Nausea and vomiting																															
Diarrhea																															
Constipation																															
Hot and cold																															
Faintness, dizziness																															
Fatigue																															
Headaches																															
Congestive Cramping																															
Dull, aching pain in pelvic region																															
Backache																															
Bloating																															
Weight gain																															
Breast tenderness																															
Headaches																															
Irritability																															
Secondary Cramping																															
Pelvic pain																															
Back pain																															
Spotting																															
Pain during/after intercourse																															
Puslike vaginal discharge																															
Fever, chills																															
Urinary frequency																															
Bowel changes																															

today. Then read over the next section on risk factors and evaluations to see which of your habits are contributing to your cramps. This will make it easier to pick specific treatments for your symptoms and devise a personalized treatment program as outlined in the later self-help sections in the book. After that, you may want to keep making monthly calendars to check your progress.

RISK FACTORS FOR MENSTRUAL CRAMPS

You are at higher risk of menstrual cramps if you have any of the factors listed below. Make a list of each risk factor that applies to you.

Use of tampons
Use of IUD
Recurrent bladder infections
Recurrent yeast infections
Childlessness (PSD)
Multiple pregnancies (PCD)
Endometriosis
Fibroid tumors
Pelvic inflammatory disease (PID)
Lack of exercise

Poor posture
Emotional stress
Daily use of:
  Salt
  Animal fats
  Dairy products
  Wheat
  Alcohol
  Sugar

Eating Habits
All foods listed below as high-stress foods can worsen cramps. If you eat a substantial number of them, or if you eat any of them frequently, your nutritional habits may be significantly contributing to your symptoms. It is best to limit or eliminate entirely your intake of all these foods.

All the foods listed under high-nutrient, low-stress foods may help relieve or prevent cramp symptoms. Include them frequently in your diet.

Make a list of the foods you eat and the frequency with which you eat them: never, once a month, once a week, twice a week or more.

High-Stress Foods
Cow's milk
Cow's cheese

Wheat-based flour
Pastries

Butter
Ice cream
Eggs
Chocolate
Sugar
Alcohol
Beef
Pork
Lamb
Wheat bread
Wheat noodles

Added salt
Bouillon
Commercial salad dressing
Catsup
Coffee
Black tea
Soft drinks
Hot dogs
Ham
Bacon

High-Nutrient, Low-Stress Foods

Avocado
Beans
Broccoli
Brussels sprouts
Cabbage
Carrots
Celery
Collards
Cucumbers
Eggplant
Garlic
Horseradish
Kale
Lettuce
Mustard greens
Okra
Onions
Parsnips
Peas
Potatoes

Radishes
Spinach
Squash
Sweet potatoes
Tomatoes
Turnips
Turnip greens
Yams
Brown rice
Millet
Barley
Oatmeal
Buckwheat
Rye
Raw flax seeds
Corn
Raw pumpkin seeds
Raw sesame seeds
Raw sunflower seeds
Raw almonds

Raw filberts
Raw pecans
Raw walnuts
Apples
Bananas
Berries
Pears
Seasonal fruits
Corn oil
Flax oil
Olive oil
Sesame oil
Safflower oil
Poultry
Fish

Exercise Habits

Exercise helps prevent cramps by relaxing muscles and promoting better blood circulation and oxygenation to the pelvic area. It can also help reduce stress and relieve anxiety. If you exercise less than three times a week, you will probably be more prone to cramp symptoms. See the sections on various kinds of exercise that can help relieve and prevent symptoms.

If you are exercising more than three times a week, keep it up.

You may want to add specific corrective exercises, choosing them to fit your symptoms.

List the frequency with which you do any of the following: never, once a month, once a week, twice a week or more.

Walking   Dancing   Bicycling   Stretching
Running   Swimming   Tennis   Yoga

Stress Evaluation Tool

If you are experiencing any of the following life events, list those that apply to you.

Death of spouse or close family member
Divorce from spouse
Death of a close friend
Legal separation from spouse
Loss of job
Radical loss of financial security
Major personal injury or illness (gynecologic or other cause)
Future surgery for gynecologic or other illness
Beginning a new marriage
Foreclosure of mortgage or loan
Lawsuit lodged against you
Marriage reconciliation
Change in health of a family member
Major trouble with boss or co-workers
Increase in responsibility — at job or home
Sexual harassment, rape or wife battering
Learning you are pregnant
Difficulties with your sexual abilities
Gaining a new family member
Change to a different job
Increase in number of marital arguments
New loan or mortgage of more than $100,000
Son or daughter leaving home
Major disagreement with in-laws or friends
Spouse begins or stops work
Recognition for outstanding achievements
Begin or end education
Undergo a change in living conditions
Revise or alter your personal habits
Change in work hours or conditions
Change of residence

Change your school or major in school
Alterations in your recreational activities
Change in church or club activities
Change in social activities
Change in sleeping habits
Change in number of family get-togethers
Diet or eating habits are changed
You go on vacation
The year-end holidays occur
You commit a minor violation of the law

Listing many items in the first third of this scale indicates major life stress and possible vulnerability to serious illness. The more items listed in the first two-thirds, the higher your stress quotient. Do everything possible to manage your stress in a healthy way. Eat the foods that provide a high-nutrient, low-stress diet, exercise on a regular basis and learn methods of stress reduction and deep breathing.

If you list fewer items, you are probably at lower risk for illness. Because stresses too minimal to include in this evaluation may also play a part in increasing your cramps, you will still benefit from practicing stress reduction techniques. Stress management is very important in helping you gain control over muscle tension.

Daily Stress Evaluation

Not all stresses have a major impact on our lives; most of us experience a multitude of small life stresses on a daily basis. The effects of these stresses are cumulative and can be a major factor in triggering muscle tension in the pelvic area on an unconscious basis. List each item that applies to you.

Work
• Too much responsibility. Too many demands are made on you. You worry about getting all your work done and doing it well.
• Time urgency. You always feel rushed. There are not enough hours in the day to complete your work.
• Job instability. There are layoffs at your company and much insecurity and concern among your fellow employees.
• Job performance. You don't feel you are working up to your maximum capability because of outside stresses. You are unhappy with your performance and therefore worried about job security.
• Difficulty getting along with boss and co-workers. Your boss is

too picky, critical and demanding. You must work closely with difficult co-workers
• Understimulation. Work is boring and makes you tired. You wish you were somewhere else.
• Uncomfortable physical conditions. Lights are too bright or dim; noises are too loud; you are exposed to noxious fumes or chemicals. You find it hard to concentrate with too much activity around you.

Spouse or Significant Other
• Hostile communication. There is too much negative emotion and drama. You are always upset or angry.
• Not enough communications. You both tend to hold in your feelings and not discuss issues. An emotional bond is lacking between you.
• Discrepancy in communications. One person talks about feelings too much, the other too little.
• Affection. There is not enough holding, touching and loving in your relationship. Or you are uncomfortable with your partner's demands for affection.
• Sexuality. There is not enough sexual intimacy and you feel deprived. Or your partner demands sex too often.
• Children. They make too much noise and too many demands on you. They are hard to discipline.
• Organization. Home is always messy; chores are half-finished.
• Time. There is too much to do and never enough time to do it all.
• Responsibility. Too many demands are made on you. You need more help.

Your Emotional State
• Too much anxiety. You constantly worry about every little thing and about what can go wrong.
• Victimization. Everyone takes advantage of you or wants to hurt you.
• Poor self-image. You are always finding fault with yourself.
• Too critical. You are always finding fault with others rather than seeing their good sides.
• Inability to relax. You are always tense, restless and wound up.
• Not enough self-renewal. You don't play enough or take enough time off to relax and have fun.
• Too angry. Small life issues upset you unduly. You become

easily angry and irritable with your husband, children, co-workers or clients.

Read over the day-to-day stresses that you find difficult to handle. How many items have you listed? Becoming aware of them is the first step toward lessening their effects on your life. Methods for reducing them and helping your body deal with them are in the section on stress reduction.

How Stress Affects Your Body
This evaluation should help you become aware of where stress localizes in your body. Each woman accumulates stress differently, tensing and contracting sets of muscles in a pattern that is unique to her. For instance, storing tension in the low back and pelvic area can worsen cramps, while storing it in the neck can cause headaches. When you feel tension building up in these areas, begin deep breathing or use one of the other methods in the section on stress reduction, which will help release muscle tension rapidly. List the places where tension most commonly localizes in your body.

Low back	Chest	Headache
Pelvic area	Shoulders	Grinding teeth
Stomach muscles	Arms	Eyestrain
Thighs and calves	Neck and throat	

THE COMPLETE TREATMENT PROGRAM

You are now ready to put together your own self-help treatment program. The following summary chart will help you; use it in two ways. First, try all the therapies that interest you; some will make you feel better than others. Alternatively, read straight through the book to get a general overview and note the treatments you want to try. Then use the chart for an overview and quick spot work. The most important thing is to establish a regimen that works and practice it on a regular basis. This will enable you to see improvement in your health and vitality very quickly.

Complete Treatment Chart

Nutrition	Dietary principles: avoid dairy products, eggs, red meat, chocolate, coffee, soft drinks, alcohol, salt, sugar
Vitamins & Minerals	Optimal supplementation, with emphasis on vitamins B3, B6 and C, calcium, magnesium, potassium, zinc, essential fatty acids
Herbs	Ginger, ginkgo biloba, white willow bark, red raspberry leaf, cramp bark, chamomile, hops, chaste tree berry, dong quai, penny root
Stress Reduction	1-6
Breathing Exercises	1-4
Physical Exercise	1-5
Yoga	1-7
Acupressure Massage	1-3
Medication	Aspirin, Advil, Midol, Pamprin, Nuprin, Naprosyn, Anaprox, Ponstel, Motrin, Tylenol with codeine, Darvon, Valium, birth control pills, Danazol, Lupron

DIETARY PRINCIPLES

A healthy diet is the cornerstone of a good anti-cramp self-care program. I've found that good nutritional habits bring more relief from cramps than any other single factor. Many women, even those with severe cramps, report a noticeable decrease in pain and discomfort within one to two menstrual cycles and a greater sense of energy and well-being than they've had in years. Seemingly unrelated allergies and poor digestive function are cleared up, too.

The list of foods that worsen cramps and should be avoided may surprise you. It contains not only junk foods that are stressful to the body but foods that are staples of the American diet. Luckily, the list of foods that help relieve and prevent cramps is a long one. Once you eat more healthful foods, you'll find they are just as delicious, convenient and easy to prepare as the foods you are now eating.

FOODS THAT HELP TREAT OR PREVENT CRAMPS

Although your symptoms are limited to the days leading up to menstruation, it's best to eat the foods listed below throughout the entire month.

Whole Grains

Eat whole grains such as millet, oats, rice and rye (some women can't tolerate 100% rye). These grains are excellent sources of the following nutrients: magnesium, which helps reduce neuromuscular tension, thereby decreasing cramps; calcium, which relaxes muscle contraction; and potassium, which has a diuretic effect, reducing bloating or excessive fluid retention of PCD. (Vitamins and minerals will be thoroughly discussed in the next section.)

It may come as a surprise, but you may need to avoid wheat, which contains gluten that is difficult to digest and can be highly allergenic. Try a wheat-free diet to see if you feel better. If you do, you may want to eliminate oats and rye, since they contain some gluten. You may feel best eating buckwheat, corn and rice and rotating them every few days.

Whole grains have other benefits because of their bran or fiber content. Bran helps get rid of excess fluid, and fiber helps prevent both constipation and diarrhea. Whole grains also help bind fat and remove it from the body, and oat and rice bran are especially good at lowering cholesterol. They may also help prevent cancer of the breast, uterus, ovaries and colon (linked to diets high in animal fat). Whole grains are excellent sources of B-complex vitamins and vitamin E, which help combat fatigue and depressive symptoms. They are also excellent sources of protein, particularly when combined with beans and peas.

Whole Grain Foods

Many grocery stores and most health food stores stock whole grain cereals, breads, crackers, pancake mix and pasta. (Check brands to make sure they're not made with sugar.) Puffed millet, corn and rice and unsweetened granola are good cold breakfast cereals, while cream of rice, buckwheat groats, brown rice, millet and slow-cooking oatmeal (the quick-cooking kind is a refined grain) are excellent hot cereals. Rye crackers are a good source of potassium, and brown rice cakes are tasty with soy spreads, tuna salad or fruit and nut spreads. Concentrated sweeteners such as maple syrup, honey and applesauce can be used in small amounts on buckwheat, rice flour or triticale pancakes. Pasta made of buckwheat, rice, corn or soy is easy to digest for women with digestive symptoms and bloating.

Legumes

Beans and peas—particularly black, kidney, lima and pinto beans, chickpeas, lentils, soybeans and tofu (made from soybeans)—are excellent sources of calcium, magnesium and potassium and are high in iron, copper and zinc. Legumes are also very high in B-complex vitamins, especially B6. They are an easily used source of protein (making them an excellent substitute for meat), and they provide all the essential amino acids when eaten with grains (good combinations are rice and beans or corn bread and split pea soup). Like grains, legumes are a good source of fiber and can help normalize bowel function (though they may cause gas in some women; if so, take digestive enzymes and eat small quantities). Because they are digested slowly, they help regulate blood sugar levels, making them ideal for women with diabetes or blood sugar imbalances.

Vegetables

Many vegetables are high in calcium, magnesium and potassium, which help relieve and prevent PSD. Both calcium and magnesium act as natural tranquilizers, helping to relax tense muscles and calm emotions. Potassium also aids in relieving PCD, reducing fluid retention and bloating. Some of the best sources of these minerals are beet and mustard greens, broccoli, green beans, kale, peas, potatoes, spinach, sweet potatoes and Swiss chard.

Many vegetables are high in vitamin C, an important antistress vitamin needed for healthy adrenal hormone production. Vitamin C boosts immune function and wound healing and its anti-infectious properties may help reduce bladder and vaginal infections, which can cause secondary dysmenorrhea. Vegetables high in vitamin C include broccoli, Brussels sprouts, cauliflower, kale, parsley, peas, peppers, potatoes and tomatoes.

Fruits

Fruits contain a wide range of nutrients, including bioflavonoids and vitamin C, essential for good circulation in tense pelvic muscles. Berries, grapefruits, oranges and melons are the best sources of vitamin C. All fruits are excellent sources of potassium, but figs, raisins and bananas are the best, so they should be eaten by women with fatigue and bloating. Certain fruits are good sources of calcium and magnesium, including bananas, blackberries, dried figs, oranges and raisins.

Eat fruits whole to take advantage of their high-fiber content, which helps prevent constipation and other digestive irregularities. Don't worry that fruit is high in sugar; its high-fiber content helps slow down absorption of the sugar and stabilizes blood sugar levels. Fresh and dried fruits make excellent snack and dessert substitutes. Use fruit juices only in small quantities. Because juice does not contain the fiber of the whole fruit, it acts more like refined table sugar and can destabilize your blood sugar level.

Seeds and Nuts

Seeds and nuts are the best sources of essential fatty acids needed to produce series-one muscle-relaxant prostaglandins. The best sources are raw flax, pumpkin, sesame and sunflower seeds. Seeds and nuts are also very high in magnesium, calcium and potassium and are excellent sources of B-complex vitamins and vitamin E, which help combat stress and regulate hormone balance. Sesame and sunflower seeds, almonds, pecans and pistachios are particularly good, but only in small quantities, because they are very high in calories.

The oils in seeds and nuts are perishable, so avoid exposure to light, heat and oxygen. Eat them raw and unsalted for the most benefit and remove the shells yourself. If you buy them shelled, refrigerate so the oils don't become rancid. Seeds and nuts make a wonderful garnish on salads, vegetable dishes and casseroles and can be eaten as a main source of protein with snacks and light meals.

Meat, Poultry and Fish

Eat meat only in small quantities (3 ounces or less a day) or avoid entirely. Red meats like beef, pork and lamb and poultry contain saturated fats that produce series-two prostaglandins which worsen cramps. Meat is also the main source of unhealthy saturated fats, which put you at higher risk of heart disease and cancer. If you wish, use meat more as a garnish and flavoring for casseroles, stir-fries and soups. Buying it from organic, range-fed sources cuts your exposure to pesticides, antibiotics and hormones. I recommend eating fish, particularly salmon, tuna, mackerel and trout, which contains essential fatty acids that helps relax muscles. Fish are excellent sources of minerals, especially iodine and potassium.

Oils

Use vegetable oils in small amounts for cooking, stir-frying and sautéing. Make sure the oils are cold pressed to ensure freshness and purity, and keep them refrigerated to avoid rancidity. Select oils such as soybean and corn that contain vitamin E, which helps normalize hormone levels and reduce mood symptoms, fatigue and cramps in women with fibroids. Women with fibroids should take vitamin E in both supplements and dietary sources such as wheat germ oil, which contains the highest levels of vitamin E and is the source of most natural vitamin E sold today.

FOODS TO AVOID

Dairy Products

Dairy products are the main dietary source of arachidonic acid, which produces muscle-contracting series-two prostaglandins. Dairy's high-saturated fat content promotes excess estrogen, which triggers fibroid tumors. Dairy's high salt content increases bloating and fluid retention of PCD. Dairy products have many other unhealthy effects: they may increase fatigue, lead to digestive problems like bloating, gas and bowel changes and decrease calcium and iron absorption. I've seen the severity of cramps decrease by as much as a third to a half within one cycle when women stop eating dairy products.

Women who are concerned about their calcium intake will find that beans, green leafy vegetables, peas, sesame seeds, soup stock made from chicken or fish bones and soybeans are other good sources of calcium. Excellent substitutes in cooking are potato, soy and nut milk (see list below), sold in health food stores. You can also take supplements of calcium, magnesium and vitamin D.

Fats

In the typical American diet, 40 percent of calories come from such sources of saturated fat as dairy products, red meats and eggs. These fats can intensify cramps by stimulating the production of muscle-contracting prostaglandins. They also promote fibroid tumor growth and heavy menstrual flow. Fat from animal sources also puts women at high risk for heart disease and cancer of the breast, uterus and ovaries.

Instead of eating foods high in saturated fats, eat more fruits, vegetables, grains, fish and poultry prepared with a minimum of fats and oils. Avoid packaged and processed foods with high-fat content. You can flavor foods with garlic, onions, herbs, lemon juice or a little olive oil (a monosaturated fat). Eat raw seeds and nuts sparingly because of their high fat content.

Salt

Too much dietary salt found in table salt, MSG and food additives can worsen bloating and fluid retention of PCD, increase high blood pressure and promote osteoporosis in menopausal women. Most processed foods (such as chips, cheeses and salad dressings), frozen and canned foods and fast foods contain large amounts of salt. For an anti-cramp diet it's best to eliminate salt and use seasonings such as garlic, herbs, spices and lemon juice. Read labels on all foods; if sodium (salt) content is high, don't buy the product.

Alcohol

Avoid alcohol entirely or drink only small amounts, not exceeding 4 ounces of wine, 10 ounces of beer or 1 ounce of hard liquor per day. Alcohol depletes the body's B-complex vitamins and minerals such as magnesium, intensifying muscle spasms, fatigue and mood swings. Excessive alcohol intake is associated with lack of ovulation, elevated estrogen levels (which can trigger fibroid growth and worsen fluid retention) and heavy menstrual flow.

For optimal health, use alcohol as an occasional treat, not more than once or twice a week. Mineral water with a twist of lemon or lime is a good substitute, or you can try nonalcoholic beverages like "near beer" or light wines.

Sugar

Sugar depletes the body's B-complex vitamins and minerals, which can worsen muscle and nervous tension, irritability and anxiety. Unfortunately, sugar addiction is very common in our society — the average American eats 120 pounds per year. Sugar is high in convenience foods like salad dressing and catsup, soft drinks and desserts. To satisfy your sweet tooth, eat healthier foods such as fruit or small amounts of grain-based desserts, like oatmeal cookies made with fruit or honey.

Caffeine

Coffee, black tea, soft drinks and chocolate all contain caffeine, as do over-the-counter menstrual remedies. Caffeine has many negative effects on the body: it increases anxiety, irritability and mood swings; depletes the body's stores of B-complex vitamins and essential minerals (increasing cramps and fatigue and interfering with estrogen levels); and inhibits iron absorption, worsening anemia.

HOW TO SUBSTITUTE HEALTHY INGREDIENTS IN RECIPES

Making substitutions for high-stress ingredients allows you to use your favorite recipes, retain their flavor and taste and not compromise your health. You can also totally eliminate high-stress ingredients, for example, making pizza with lots of vegetables but no cheese. Or you can cut down amounts of high-stress ingredients, for example, decreasing cow's milk cheese by one-half to two-thirds or sweetener by one-third to one-half.

Substitutes for Common High-Stress Ingredients

¾ cup sugar	½ cup honey
	¼ cup molasses
	½ cup maple syrup
	½ ounce barley malt
	1 cup apple butter
	2 cups apple juice
	Eliminate sweetener and add extra fruit and nuts to pastries
1 cup milk	1 cup soy, potato (DariFree), nut or grain milk
cheeses	Lower-fat cheeses, goat's or sheep's cheese; soy cheese in sandwiches, salads, pizzas, lasagnas and casseroles
1 tablespoon butter	1 tablespoon flax oil (must use raw, unheated; buy in health food stores or order through The LifeCycles Center)

½ teaspoon salt	1 tablespoon miso
	½ teaspoon potassium chloride salt substitute
	½ teaspoon Mrs. Dash, Spike
	½ teaspoon herbs (basil, tarragon, oregano)
	Powdered seaweeds (kelp or nori) to season vegetables, grains, salads. Add small amount of low-salt soy sauce or Bragg's Amino Acids to soups, casseroles, stir-fries at end of cooking process
1½ cups cocoa	1 cup powdered carob
1 square chocolate	¾ tablespoon powdered carob
1 tablespoon coffee	1 tablespoon decaffeinated coffee
	1 tablespoon Pero, Postum, Caffix or other grain-based coffee substitute
	Herbal teas; for morning pick-up, grate a few teaspoons of fresh ginger root into a pot of water, boil, steep and serve with honey
4 ounces wine	4 ounces light wine
8 ounces beer	8 ounces near beer
1 cup white flour	1 cup barley flour (pie crust)
	1 cup rice flour (cookies, cakes, breads)

VITAMINS, MINERALS AND HERBS

Optimal nutrition plays a crucial role in both treatment and prevention of cramps. Nutrients help relieve cramps by promoting normal hormone production and balance, muscle tone and relaxation in the pelvis and lower back, and good blood circulation. When adequate nutritional support is lacking, it's very difficult to relieve symptoms, even with powerful drugs. In fact, poor or inadequate nutrition may play a major role in causing cramp symptoms.

The importance of supplementing a good diet with nutrients cannot be emphasized too strongly. (However, taking supplements does not excuse poor nutritional habits.) It's hard for most women to get their nutrient intake up to the levels needed for optimal healing through diet alone. Taking supplements corrects this deficiency and helps you heal rapidly and completely.

VITAMINS AND MINERALS

Where possible, I have included optimal doses for the nutrients described below. Lower doses may work better for you, so start slowly and increase your dose gradually to find the best level for you.

Vitamin B-Complex

These vitamins consist of eleven factors that perform a number of important biochemical functions, including stabilization of brain chemistry, glucose metabolism and inactivation of estrogen by the liver. Emotional and nutritional stress causes loss of B vitamins from the body, which can worsen certain symptoms, including fatigue, faintness and dizziness. I recommend 50 to 100 mg per day of B-complex vitamins. Common food sources are blackstrap molasses, egg yolks, legumes, liver and whole grains.

Two B vitamins — B3 and B6 — are particularly useful for cramps. Research has shown that niacin, or vitamin B3, helps relieve 90% of menstrual cramps; its effectiveness is enhanced with vitamin C and rutin. Start taking 25 to 200 mg per day seven to ten days prior to your period to be effective. (Women with preexisting liver disease should use B3 cautiously.)

Vitamin B6, or pyridoxine, helps regulate symptoms of both PSD and PCD. Studies have shown it helps reduce cramping, fatigue, fluid retention and weight gain. Vitamin B6 is also an important factor in the production of beneficial series-one prostaglandins, which have a relaxant effect on uterine muscles. B6 can be safely used in doses up to 300 mg, but not higher. Good food sources are chicken, salmon, shrimp, sunflower seeds, tuna, whole grains and vegetables, especially asparagus, broccoli, cauliflower, green peas, leeks and sweet potatoes.

Vitamin C

Vitamin C helps increase capillary permeability, which permits better flow of nutrients into the tight, contracted uterine muscle and of waste products out of the uterus. Vitamin C also counteracts stress and helps decrease symptoms of fatigue and lethargy. I recommend from 500 to 3000 mg daily, especially with symptoms. Good sources of vitamin C are fruits, including all citrus fruits, berries, cantaloupes, kiwis and pineapples; most vegetables, but especially asparagus, broccoli, cabbage, collards, potatoes, tomatoes and turnips; and all types of liver, pheasant, quail and salmon.

Vitamin E

Studies have shown that taking vitamin E helps relieve symptoms of PSD within two menstrual cycles in approximately 70% of the women tested. Vitamin E has a powerful effect on the hormonal system and has been used to reduce breast tenderness, fibrocystic breast diseases and PMS symptoms, as well as hot flashes in menopausal women. The best natural sources of vitamin E are wheat germ, walnut, soybean and other grain and seed oils as well as almonds, asparagus, brown rice, cucumbers, haddock, herring, lamb, mangoes, millet, peanuts and all types of liver. I recommend 400 to 800 I.U. per day, though women with hypertension and diabetes should start at a much lower dosage (100 I.U./day) and any increase should be monitored slowly and carefully.

Calcium

This mineral helps prevent cramps by maintaining normal muscle tone. When taken before bed, it also helps combat insomnia. Calcium is a major structural component of bones and prevents osteoporosis. Unfortunately, calcium deficiency is common in our society, with the typical American diet supplying only 450 to 550 mg per day. The recommended daily allowance (RDA) for calcium in menstruating women is 800 mg per day and rises to as much as 1500 mg per day in postmenopausal women. Good food sources of calcium include blackstrap molasses, green leafy vegetables, legumes, seafood, whole grains and fruits, including berries, oranges, prunes and raisins.

Magnesium

Magnesium has an important effect in reducing cramps through the neuromuscular system. A magnesium deficiency worsens menstrual fatigue, dizziness, fainting and retards the conversion of essential fatty acids to beneficial series-one prostaglandins. Like calcium, magnesium is a structural component of healthy bone tissue and is needed to prevent osteoporosis. Because magnesium and calcium work together—magnesium optimizes the amount of usable calcium in the body by increasing calcium absorption—it is recommended that the diet include half as much magnesium as calcium, or about 400 mg per day. Most women get only one-third to one-half that amount in their daily diet. Good sources of magnesium include meat, nuts and seeds, poultry, seafood, whole grains, fruits, especially avocados, bananas, papayas, prunes and raisins, and vegetables like artichokes, corn, green peas, potatoes, spinach, squash and yams

Iron

Women who have iron deficiency anemia may be at higher risk of cramps because of the lower oxygen-carrying capability of their red blood cells. One study showed that cramping disappeared when iron deficiency anemia was cured. Young women in their teens and twenties who eat an iron-poor diet are not only very prone to iron deficiency, but at the peak age for PSD. Good food sources of iron include blackstrap molasses, eggs, leafy green vegetables, legumes, liver, seafood, seeds and nuts, whole grains and fruits, especially avocados, blackberries, and dried dates, figs, prunes and raisins. The RDA for iron is 15 mg.

HERBS

A wide variety of herbs are gentle, effective remedies for alleviating cramp symptoms. They provide extended nutrition and are a way of balancing and expanding the diet and optimizing nutritional intake. Some herbs provide an additional source of essential nutrients such as calcium, magnesium and potassium; others have mild relaxant, diuretic and anti-inflammatory properties. In Asian medicine, cramps are considered a *yang* condition, worsened by meat and salt which have a contracting effect on the body. Cramps are treated by special herbs that have a *yin* effect, causing muscle relaxation and blood vessel dilation.

Sedative Herbs

Chamomile, hops, passion flower and valerian root have a significant calming effect on the central nervous system and promote muscle relaxation as well as emotional calm and well-being. Take them for restful sleep and help in combating insomnia. You can make soothing teas of chamomile, hops and peppermint; since valerian has an unpleasant taste, take it in capsule form.

Muscle-Relaxant Herbs

Several Asian herbs—notably Dong Quai, or angelica sinensis, and peony root—have been used for thousands of years to cure cramps; they directly relax the uterine muscle. You can buy them in health food stores and Asian herbal shops. Angelica root also has pain-relieving properties, rivaling aspirin. Several native American herbs, including black cohosh, black haw bark, cramp bark and unicorn root, are also effective. For instance, cramp bark contains high doses of vitamin C, which helps relax cramped muscles.

Anti-Inflammatory Herbs

Both meadowsweet and white willow bark, which has a long and distinguished history as an effective pain reliever in both Eastern and Western healing traditions, reduce inflammation, pain and fever so they can be used effectively to treat cramps and headaches. The active painkilling chemical in both herbs is salicylic acid, which is the precursor of aspirin. Unfortunately, like aspirin, they can produce unwanted side effects of gastric indigestion, nausea and diarrhea, so use them carefully.

Diuretic Herbs

Since many herbs act as mild diuretic agents, they are useful in reducing bloating and fluid retention of PCD. Some of the most commonly used, in mild teas or tinctures, are buchu, celery, dandelion, horsetail, nettle, parsley, sarsaparilla and uva ursi. Because they can deplete your potassium stores over time, be sure to eat foods that are high in potassium such as bananas, oranges, raw seeds and nuts, as well as most fruits and fresh vegetables.

Blood-Circulation Enhancers

Certain herbs such as ginger and ginkgo biloba improve circulation to the pelvis and lower extremities. Ginger also has an antispasmodic effect and can help relieve digestive symptoms, including nausea, vomiting and bowel changes. Besides taking ginger in tincture or capsule form, you can also drink it as a delicious tea (for instructions, see chart on substitutes above). You can also combine the two herbs effectively.

ESSENTIAL FATTY ACIDS

Sufficient essential fatty acids are an extremely important part of any anti-cramp program. As discussed above, essential fatty acids—both linoleic (Omega 6 family) and linolenic acid (Omega 3 family)—are the raw materials from which beneficial series-one prostaglandins are made. They help promote muscle and blood-vessel relaxation that significantly reduce cramps and tension. Fatty acids are derived from raw nuts, seeds and certain cold-water, high-fat fish. Good sources are flax, sesame and sunflower seeds and wheat germ; corn, safflower, sesame seed, soybean, sunflower, walnut and wheat germ oils; and eel, mackerel, rainbow trout, salmon and tuna. They cannot be made by the body but must be supplied daily from either food or supplements. The average healthy adult requires only four teaspoons per day, though women with cramps may need up to several tablespoons. For optimal results, be sure to use these oils along with vitamin E (which also helps prevent rancidity).

Some women may lack the ability to efficiently convert fatty acids to prostaglandins, which requires the presence of magnesium, niacin, vitamins B6 and C and zinc. This is especially true for women who eat a high-cholesterol diet, processed oils such as mayonnaise, use a great deal of alcohol or are diabetic. Other factors that impede prostaglandin production include allergies, eczema and emotional stress. The rest of the fatty acids can be used as an energy source, but they don't play a role in relieving cramp symptoms.

A number of studies have shown that essential fatty acids can reduce most PMS symptoms by as much as 70%. (Women with PMS often have PCD.) Evening primrose, black currant and borage oils are the most common supplements used to treat cramps and PMS.

The best food sources of essential fatty acids are raw flax seed and pumpkin seed oils. Both the seeds and their pressed oils can be used and should be absolutely fresh and unspoiled. Because these oils become rancid very easily when exposed to light and air (oxygen), they need to be packed in special opaque containers and refrigerated. Fresh flax seed oil is my special favorite. Its golden, rich, delicious flavor makes it an ideal butter replacement. The only restriction when using flax oil is not to heat or cook it, because that damages its chemical properties. (If you use the whole flax seed, remember that the seeds are 50 percent oil by content, so you need twice as much whole seed intake as oil to obtain the same amount of fatty acids.) Because pumpkin seed oil is hard to find, eating fresh raw pumpkin seeds is a good source of this oil. Both oils can also be taken in capsule form.

NUTRITIONAL SUPPLEMENTS

The following formulas provide excellent nutritional support for both PSD and PCD and are typical of those I use with patients. It's best if you put together your own individualized program. Be sure to take all supplements with meals or snacks. If you have a digestive reaction, such as nausea or indigestion, stop all supplements, then start again, adding one at a time until you find the offending nutrient and eliminate it from your program. If you have questions, consult a health-care professional who is knowledgeable about nutrition.

Remember that all women differ somewhat in their nutritional needs. Start with one-quarter to one-half of the dose recommended and slowly work your way up to a higher level. Most women may want to take smaller doses when they are symptom-free; two or three capsules per day may be enough. Then when your symptoms occur, double the dose. *Caution:* Do not exceed six to eight capsules per day without your doctor's supervision.

Optimal Nutritional Supplementation (daily doses)

VITAMINS	
Beta-carotene	15,000 I.U.
Biotin	30 mcg
Choline bitartrate, inositol	500 mg
Folic acid	200 mcg
Vitamins B1 (thiamine), B2, B3 (niacinamide), B12, pantothenic acid, PABA (para-aminobenzoic acid)	50 mg
Vitamin B6 (pyridoxine HCl)	100 mg
Vitamin C	1,000 mg
Vitamin D (cholecalciferol)	100 I.U.
Vitamin E	600 I.U.
MINERALS	
Calcium (amino acid chelate)	150 mg
Magnesium	300 mg

Chromium	100 mcg
Copper	0.5 mg
Iodine	150 mcg
Iron (amino acid chelate)	15 mg
Manganese	10 mg
Potassium	100 mg
Selenium	25 mcg
Zinc	25 mg

Optimal Herbal Supplements (daily doses based on herbal tinctures)

Ginger root, white willow bark	200 mg
Chamomile, cramp bark, hops, sarsaparilla	150 mg

STRESS REDUCTION

To feel rushed and tense is typical given the pace of our goal-oriented culture. The resulting emotional stress can be a significant trigger for pain, discomfort and muscle tension. My patients often tell me their cramps are worse when they are more upset. Though we can't avoid stress today, we can modify its physical and psychological effects.

As your period approaches, I recommend using a variety of stress-reduction techniques, including focusing, meditation, affirmations and visualizations, on a daily basis. You can also try taking a 20-minute warm bath, listening to classical music or nature sounds and biofeedback therapy (available at many hospitals, universities and stress management clinics).

In preparation, dress in loose clothing, and find a comfortable position, keeping your spine straight and your arms and legs uncrossed. Focus your attention fully on the exercises. Close your eyes and take a few deep breaths to take your thoughts off the day's activities.

Try each of the following exercises at least once. Experiment until you find the combination that works for you. Ideally, you should do the exercises at least a few minutes each day.

Exercise 1: Focusing
This exercise takes your attention off the pelvic region and lower part of your body and focuses it elsewhere.
- Sit upright in a comfortable position. Hold several coins, such as two quarters, in the palm of your hands. Focus all your attention on them.
- Inhale and exhale, continuing to concentrate for 30 seconds. Don't let any other thoughts intrude. Then, notice your breathing. It is probably slower and calmer. You will probably feel a sense of peace and less anxiety and physical discomfort.

Exercise 2: Progressive Muscle Relaxation
This exercise will help you locate areas of muscle tension and release them. This helps relieve tight muscles that women with cramps, low back pain and abdominal discomfort have at all times. Tensing pelvic muscles is an unconscious response to many work, relationship and sexual stresses that develop over time and sets up the emotional patterning that triggers cramps. Movement is an effective way to break these habits.
- Lie on your back in a comfortable position with your arms resting at your sides, palms down.
- Inhale and exhale slowly and deeply. Clench your hands into fists, hold them tight for 15 seconds and relax the rest of your body. Visualize (imagine in your mind) your fists contracting, becoming tighter and tighter.
- Relax your hands. As you relax, see a golden light flowing into your entire body, making all your muscles soft and pliable.
- Tense and relax the following parts of your body in this order: face, shoulders, back, stomach, pelvis, legs, feet and toes. Hold each part tensed for 15 seconds and then relax your body for 30 seconds before going on to the next part.
- Finish the exercise by shaking your hands and imagining any remaining tension flowing out your fingertips.

Exercise 3: Healing Meditation
The exercise is based on the premise that the mind and the body are linked. When you visualize a beautiful scene in which your body is being healed, you actually stimulate positive chemical and hormonal changes in your body that help create this condition. I

have seen the power of positive thinking for years in my medical practice. Meditations can be a powerful tool for healing.

- Lie on your back in a comfortable position. Inhale and exhale slowly and deeply.
- Visualize a beautiful green meadow full of lovely fragrant flowers. In the middle of the meadow is a golden temple. See it emanating peace and healing.
- Visualize yourself entering this temple alone. It is still and peaceful. You feel a healing energy filling every pore of your body with a warm golden light. This energy is a healing balm that totally relaxes you. All anxiety dissolves from your mind. You feel at ease.
- Open your eyes and continue breathing deeply and slowly for a few more cycles.

Exercise 4. Peaceful Meditation

You can adapt the healing meditation to reduce stress. Just focus all your attention on your breathing and say the word "peace" as you inhale. Say the word "calm" as you exhale, drawing out the words so they last the entire breath.

Exercise 5: Affirmations

Affirmations align your mind with your body in a positive way through the power of suggestion. In addition to following an excellent diet and vigorous exercise routine, you must develop a positive belief system and body image.

While sitting in a comfortable position, repeat the following affirmations, saying the ones that are important to you three times. Feel free to add affirmations that are meaningful to you.

- My female system is strong and healthy.
- My hormones are balanced, normal and perfectly regulated.
- My body chemistry is balanced and normal.
- I am relaxed and at ease as my period approaches.
- I go through my monthly menstrual cycle with ease.
- I feel wonderful each month before I menstruate.
- My uterus is relaxed and receptive; I welcome my period.
- My low back muscles feel supple and pliable with each cycle.
- I desire a well-balanced and healthful diet.
- I eat only the foods that are good for my body.
- It is a real pleasure to take good care of my body.
- I love my body and feel at ease with it.
- I handle stress easily and in a relaxed manner.

Exercise 6: Visualizations

Visualization is a powerful imaging technique that can actually stimulate positive chemical and hormonal changes in your body and help create the desired outcome. You are literally imaging your body the way you want it to be. Its use was pioneered by Carl Simonton, M.D., a cancer radiation therapist, who had his patients imagine their immune systems as big white knights destroying small, insignificant cancer cells. Visualization exercises can also help modify your behavior so you are more likely to choose foods carefully and follow regular exercise programs to help your body fit the images you desire.

Visualizing the following scene should take a minute or two. Linger on any images that particularly please you.

- Close your eyes. Begin to breathe deeply, inhaling and exhaling slowly. Feel your body begin to relax.
- Imagine that you can look deep inside your body. Look at your female organs. See that your uterus is relaxed, supple and has good blood circulation bringing it nourishment and taking away wastes. See that your ovaries are healthy and produce just the right level of hormones. See that your fallopian tubes, which carry eggs to your ovaries, are totally open, elastic and healthy.
- Look at your abdominal and low back muscles. See that they have healthy muscle tone; see them relaxed during your period. See that your fluid balance is perfect in your pelvic area.
- Look at your entire body and enjoy the sense of peace and calm radiating through it.
- Stop visualizing and focus on slow, deep breathing. Open your eyes and feel very good.

BREATHING EXERCISES

The whole body needs optimal levels of oxygen for building, repair and elimination. When you have cramps, you tend to tense your muscles, constrict blood flow, elevate your pulse rate and heartbeat and stimulate the output of stressful chemicals from your glands. Harmful waste products accumulate in your muscles and other tissues. Therapeutic breathing exercises break up this pattern and help the body return to equilibrium.

Exercise 1: Deep Abdominal Breathing

Deep, slow abdominal breathing brings adequate oxygen to all tissues, helps relax the entire body and calm many other physiological processes, such as rapid pulse rate and heartbeat that often accompany cramps.

- Lie flat on your back with your knees pulled up and your feet slightly apart. Breathe in and out through your nose.
- Inhale deeply, allowing your stomach to balloon out. Visualize your lungs filling up with air so your chest swells out.
- Imagine the air you breathe is filling your body with energy.
- Exhale deeply, letting your stomach and chest collapse.

Exercise 2: Peaceful, Slow Breathing

You can adapt deep abdominal breathing to reduce stress. Just imagine that the air you are breathing is filled with peace and calm and repeat the sequence until you feel relaxed.

Exercise 3: Grounding Breath

Women in pain and discomfort often lose the sense of being grounded, which makes it very difficult to function mentally. This exercise will help you focus both physically and mentally.

- Sit upright in a chair in a comfortable position, with your feet slightly apart. Breathe in and out through your nose.
- Inhale deeply, allowing your stomach to balloon out. Visualize your lungs filling up with air so your chest swells out. Hold your inhalation.
- See a large, thick cord running from the bottom of your buttocks to the center of the earth. Follow the cord all the way down and see it fastened securely to the earth's center. Run two smaller cords from the bottom of your feet down to the center of the earth.
- As you exhale, gently push your buttocks into the seat of your chair. Become aware of your buttocks, thighs, calves, ankles and feet. Feel their strength and solidity.
- Repeat this exercise several times until you feel fully grounded.

Exercise 4: Muscle Tension Release Breathing

A woman with cramps can have tight, tense muscles in other parts of her body and not be aware of it. This exercise will help you focus on any tension you are carrying in your upper body and take your focus off your cramps. It will also help release muscle tension in your entire body. This is a good exercise to do while walking or doing sports or desk work.

- Sit upright in a chair in a comfortable position, with your feet slightly apart. Breathe in and out through your nose.
- Inhale and exhale deeply, moving your head from side to side. Keep your shoulders down and try to touch your ear to your shoulder. Imagine that your neck is made out of putty so it moves in a supple, relaxed manner.
- Now inhale and pull your shoulders toward your ears. Hold your breath and keep your shoulders hunched. Exhale and let your shoulders drop to a relaxed position. Repeat several times.
- Inhale and exhale deeply as you roll your shoulders forward in a large, slow, circular motion. Then roll your shoulders back slowly. Repeat several times.
- Inhale and exhale deeply, keeping the rest of your body still and relaxed. Repeat several times.

PHYSICAL EXERCISE

Exercise promotes pain relief and prevention of cramps for a number of reasons. Tight, tense uterine and back muscles have decreased blood flow and oxygenation. Waste products like excessive carbon dioxide accumulate and can worsen symptoms. Pain causes women to contract their muscles involuntarily, and breathing may become rapid and shallow so less oxygen is taken in through respiration, further decreasing oxygen in the pelvic region. Metabolism of the muscles becomes less efficient, and fluid retention can become a problem in the pelvic area, ankles and feet.

Vigorous aerobic exercise such as tennis, walking, swimming and dancing requires deep breathing and active movement. Oxygenation and blood flow to the pelvic area improve with better respiration. The vigorous pumping action of the muscles in these activities helps reduce PCD symptoms by removing blood and other fluids from the pelvic region.

Exercise also provides significant psychological benefits. Improved oxygenation and blood flow promote optimal functioning of the brain. Exercise also helps trigger increased output of endorphins, chemicals made by the brain that have a natural opiate effect and are thought to produce the "runner's high." Many patients say vigorous exercise is their most effective form of stress management and produces a sense of peace and relaxation unmatched by anything else.

Another way that aerobic exercise helps reduce anxiety is by helping to balance the autonomic nervous system. That regulates the "fight or flight" response that many women feel around their period, when small life issues become magnified out of proportion. Regular exercise helps lessen this response.

I also recommend that women with severe cramps and low back pain do flexibility and stretching exercises. These strengthen the back and abdominal muscles, preventing these conditions.

For both prevention and treatment, I recommend a regular program of physical activity throughout the entire month. The following exercises promote mobility, flexibility and relaxation. Practiced on a regular weekly basis, they will improve vigor and energy at all times, help loosen the joints in your lower body and decrease muscle stiffness and tension during premenstrual and menstrual times of the month. A short session every day is best; if that's not possible, try every other day. I have also found many of these exercises to be very helpful during times of physical and emotional stress. Follow these guidelines:

- Do all these exercises during the first week or two of your program. Then put together your own routine, choosing the exercises that provide the most benefit. Remember that warmups should always precede any athletic events.
- Exercises should be performed in a relaxed, unhurried manner. Wear loose, comfortable clothing and work on a mat or blanket. Evacuate your bowels or bladder before you begin.
- Pay close attention to initial instructions when beginning an exercise. Visualize the exercise in your mind, then follow with proper placement of the body.
- Move slowly through the exercises to promote flexibility and prevent injury. Always rest for a few minutes afterwards.

Exercise 1: Joint Motion and Flexibility

With severe uterine cramping, women's first instinct is to curl up in a fetal position. But that is probably the worst thing you can do, because it cuts off blood flow and oxygenation to the pelvic and low back areas, worsening the pain and tension. The following sequence provides a gentle stretching of muscles around joints, helping to reduce tension and stress. These stretches are also thought to stimulate the acupuncture meridians (see later section).

- Sit on the floor with your legs together and stretched out straight in front of you, with your hands at your sides.
- *Toes:* Slowly flex and extend the toes without moving your feet or ankles. Repeat 10 times.
- *Ankles:* Slowly flex and extend the ankle joints. Repeat 10 times.
  Separate your legs slightly, then rotate your ankles in each direction 10 times. Be sure to keep your heels on the floor.
- *Knees:* Still resting in the sitting position, bend the right leg at the knee, bringing the heel near the right buttock.
  Lift the right leg off the ground, straightening the right knee. Repeat 10 times. Then do the same exercise with the left leg.
  Hold the thigh near the chest with both hands. Rotate your lower leg in a circular motion from the knee 10 times clockwise and then 10 times counterclockwise. Repeat with the left leg.
- *Hips:* Bend the left leg, placing your left foot on your right thigh. Hold the left knee with the left hand and hold the left ankle with the right hand. Then gently move the left knee up and down with the left hand. Repeat with the right leg.
  In the same position, rotate the left knee clockwise 10 times and counterclockwise 10 times. Repeat on the right side.
  Bring the soles of the feet together and the heels close to the body. Using your hands, push your knees to the floor and then let them come up. Repeat 10 times.
- *Spine:* Remain sitting with your legs together and straight in front of you. Reach over and touch your toes without bending your knees. Repeat 20 times.

Exercise 2: Muscle Tension Relaxation
This set is excellent for releasing muscle tension and improving circulation in the lower body. Many women also notice an increase in energy level. Do the steps slowly and easily so as not to cause strain or injury.

- *Legs and Pelvis:* Stand with your legs spread apart about two feet. Point your feet out at a comfortable angle. Bend your knees slowly and lower your buttocks. Eventually, they should be able to go as low as your knees. Move up and down 10 times. Now, rock your pelvis back and forth in a swinging motion.
- *Legs and Pelvis:* Move your hips and pelvis from side to side. Let your torso and arms sway in the opposite direction, as if

dancing. Then move your hips around in a full circle. Do this several times in one direction, then the other.

Exercise 3: Lower Back Arch
This exercise helps loosen the lower back muscles, promotes flexibility of the spine and combats tiredness in women who experience decreased energy during their period.
- Stand with your legs spread 1 foot apart and your feet pointing straight ahead. Place your hands around your waist with your thumbs pressing into your lower back. As you inhale, curve your back into an arch and hold your head back.
- As you exhale, let the weight of your body bend you forward so that your head almost touches your knees. Hold for a few seconds. Do this exercise slowly and repeat several times.

Exercise 4: Abdominal Muscle Release
This exercise helps release lower and upper abdominal tension and such digestive symptoms as nausea and bowel changes.
- Sit on the floor with your legs crossed. Place your hands on your shoulders with your fingers in front and your thumbs in back. Be sure to keep your spine straight and inhale deeply.
- As you inhale, twist your head, chest and abdomen to the left. As you exhale, twist your body to the right. Do this exercise 4 times. Reverse directions and repeat the sequence.

Exercise 5: Low Back Release
This exercise promotes relaxation in the lower back, hips and abdominal muscles. You may also notice a decrease in anxiety and tension.
- Lie on your back with your legs together. Raise your feet 6 to 8 inches off the ground and then raise your head and shoulders 6 inches also.
- Point to your toes with your fingertips, keeping your arms straight and your eyes fixed on your toes. Then breathe through your nose deeply to a count of 20.
- Lower your legs and head and relax for a count of 30. Repeat this exercise several times.

YOGA

Yoga's slow, controlled stretching movements help relax tense muscles and improve their suppleness and flexibility. They also help bring better blood circulation and oxygenation to the tense areas of your lower body. In addition, the deep breathing and slow movement of yoga help reduce anxiety and irritability.

The following yoga poses not only relieve cramps and discomfort, but energize and balance the female reproductive tract and help correct any underlying hormonal imbalance. Women who experience fatigue due to menstrual pain and discomfort can enjoy increased vigor and stamina when practicing these exercises.

First, read over the pose, visualizing it in your mind, then follow with the proper placement of the body. Move slowly through the pose to promote flexibility of the muscles and prevent injury. Be sure to follow the breathing instructions.

Pay close attention to the instructions when beginning an exercise. If the pose is practiced properly, you are much more likely to have relief from your symptoms. If you experience any pain or discomfort, immediately cut back until you can proceed without discomfort. If you do strain a muscle, immediately apply ice for 10 minutes to the injured area and continue use two or three times a day for several days. If the pain persists, see your doctor.

Stretch 1: Rock and Roll

This exercise helps relieve low back tension, massages the neck and spine and flexes the vertebral column, thereby reducing fatigue. Rest briefly afterwards to enhance its benefit.

- Lie on your back. Bend your knees, raising them to your chest. Interlock your fingers below your knees.
- Raise your head toward your knees and gently rock back and forth on your curved spine. Note the roundness of your back and shoulders. Keep your chin tucked in as you roll back. Avoid rolling back too far on your neck. Repeat 5 to 10 times.

Stretch 2: Pelvic Arch

This is an excellent exercise for stretching tight abdominal muscles and reducing pelvic congestion.
- Lie on your back with your knees bent. Spread your feet apart, flat on the floor. Place your hands firmly around your ankles.
- As you inhale, arch your pelvis up and hold for a few seconds. As you exhale, relax and lower your pelvis. Repeat 5 times.

Stretch 3: Cat Cow

This exercise flexes and strengthens the lower back. By building it up, you can help prevent cramps and low back pain.
- Kneel on all fours. As you inhale, arch your spine downward while your head goes back.
- As you exhale, curve your spine into a rounded arch while your head goes down. Do this exercise rhythmicly several times.

Stretch 4: The Pump

This exercise strengthens the back and abdominal muscles, improving circulation to the pelvis and calming anxiety.
- Lie down and press the small of your back into the floor. This permits you to use your abdominal muscles without straining your lower back.
- Raise your right leg slowly while breathing in, keeping your back flat on the floor and letting the rest of your body remain relaxed. Imagine your leg being pulled up smoothly by a spring. Do not jerk your leg. Hold for a few breaths. Lower your leg and breathe out.
- Repeat the same exercise on your left side. Then alternate legs 5 to 10 times.

Stretch 5: The Locust

This exercise strengthens the lower back, abdomen, buttocks and legs and helps prevent low back pain and cramps. It also energizes the entire reproductive tract.
- Lie face down on the floor. Make fists with both hands and place them under your hips. This prevents compression of the lumbar spine while doing the exercise.
- Straighten your body and raise your right leg with an upward thrust as high as you can, keeping your hips on your fists. Hold for 5 to 20 seconds, if possible.
- Lower your leg to the original position. Repeat on the left side, then with both legs together. Repeat 10 times.

Stretch 6: The Bow

This exercise stretches the entire spine and abdominal muscles and strengthens the back, hips and thighs. It also stimulates the digestive organs and endocrine glands. Regular practice helps relieve depression and fatigue.

- Lie face down on the floor, arms at your sides. Slowly bend your legs at the knees and bring your feet up toward your buttocks.
- Reach back with your arms and carefully take hold of first one foot and then the other. Flex your feet so you can grasp them more easily.
- Inhale and raise your trunk from the floor as far as possible. Lift your head and elevate your knees off the floor.
- Squeeze your buttocks. Imagine your body looking like a gently curved bow. Hold for 10 to 15 seconds.
- Slowly release the posture, allow your chin to touch the floor and finally release your feet, slowly returning them to the floor. Return to your original position. Repeat 5 times.

Stretch 7: Child's Pose

This exercise gently stretches the lower back and is excellent for relieving cramps and irritability.

- Sit on your heels. Bring your forehead to the floor, stretching the spine as far over your head as possible. Close your eyes.
- Hold for as long as it is comfortable.

ACUPRESSURE

Acupressure massage is an ancient Asian healing method in which finger pressure is applied to specific points on the body to help prevent and treat illness. Pressing specific points creates changes on two levels. Physically, acupressure affects muscle tension, blood circulation and other physiological matters. On another level, acupressure helps build the body's life energy, called chi (similar to electromagnetic energy). Health is thought to be a state in which sufficient chi is equally distributed throughout the body, energizing all the cells and tissues. Chi runs through the body in channels called meridians; disease occurs when the energy flow in a meridian is blocked. Meridian flow can be corrected by hand massage or stimulation with tiny needles (acupuncture). When the normal flow of energy is resumed, the body heals itself spontaneously.

Stimulation of acupressure points through finger pressure can be done by you or a friend following simple instructions. It is safe, painless and can be done without years of specialized training. Make sure your hands are clean and your nails trimmed. If your hands are cold, heat them with warm water.

Work on the side of the body that has the most discomfort. If both sides are equally uncomfortable, choose one. Working on one side seems to relieve symptoms on both sides.

Hold each point with steady, comfortable pressure with several fingers for one to three minutes. Apply pressure slowly with the tips of your fingers. If you feel resistance or tension, you may want to push a little harder. However, if your hand starts to feel tense or tired, lighten the pressure. If the acupressure point feels somewhat tender, it means the meridian is blocked. Tenderness should go away slowly during treatment. Some patients describe a very pleasant feeling of energy radiating out from this point into the body. Breathe gently while doing the exercises. You may massage the points once a day or more while you have symptoms.

Exercise 1: Balances the Entire Reproductive System
- *Equipment:* You will need a knotted towel to put pressure on hard-to-reach areas of the back while your hands are on other points.
- Lie on the floor with your knees up and place the towel between your shoulder blades at the top of your spine. Hold each step 1 to 3 minutes as you move the knotted towel down your spine to your waist.
- Cross your arms over your chest and press your thumbs against the inside of your upper arms.
- Now move the towel down your spine, and press your left hand at the base of your sternum (breastbone) and your right hand at the base of your head at the junction of the spine and the skull.
- Move the towel down your spine, and interlace your fingers and place them below your breasts. Press your fingertips directly against your body.
- Move the towel down your spine, and press your left hand on the top of your pubic bone and your right hand on your tailbone.

Exercise 2: Relieves Cramps, Fluid Retention, Weight Gain
This sequence balances points on the spleen meridian.
- Sit up and prop your back against a chair, or lie down and put your lower legs over the seat of a chair. Hold each step 1 to 3 minutes.
- Press your left hand in the crease of the groin where you bend your leg, one-third to one-half way between the hip bone and the outside edge of the pubic bone, and keep it there throughout the exercise. Press your right hand on a spot 2 to 3 inches above the knee.
- Move your right hand to the point below the inner part of the knee. To find the point, follow the curve of the bone just below the knee. Press the underside of the curve with your fingers.
- Move your right hand to the inside of your shin and press it. To find this point, go four fingerwidths above the ankle bone. The point is just above the top finger.
- Move your right hand to the edge of your instep and press it. To find the point, follow the big toe bone until you hit a knobby, prominent small bone.
- Move your right hand to the front and back of the big toe over the nail and press it.

Exercise 3: Relieves Low Back Pain and Cramps
This exercise balances points on the bladder meridian and the energy of the reproductive tract.
- Sit on the floor and prop your back against a wall or a heavy piece of furniture. Hold each step 1 to 3 minutes. Alternative position: Lie on the floor and put your lower legs over the seat of a chair.
- Press your right hand 1 inch above your waist on the muscle to the right side of the spine (the muscle will feel firm and ropelike), and keep it there throughout the exercise. Press your left hand behind the crease of your right knee.
- Move your left hand to the center of the back of your right calf and press. This is just below the fullest part of the calf.
- Move your left hand just below your ankle bone on the outside of the right heel and press.
- Move your left hand to the front and back of your right little toe at the nail and press.

TREATING CRAMPS WITH DRUGS

Women can choose many different types of medications to treat cramps (see chart).

Symptoms	Medication	Comments
Mild	Over the counter: asprin, ibuprofen (Advil, Nuprin) Combination (Midol, Pamprin)	Take with food to avoid upset stomach May make jittery or drowsy
Severe: PSD & endometriosis	Prescription: Prostaglandin inhibitors (Motrin, Anaprox, Ponstel, Naprosyn) Narcotics (Codeine, Darvon) Diuretics (HydroDiuril, Hygroton) Relaxants (Valium)	10% of users report digestive & other side effects Addictive Side effects & don't reverse underyling causes
Endometriosis & fibroid tumors	Hormonal therapies: birth control pills, Danazol, Lupron	Only under doctor's supervision